Avoid the Big C – Amazing Programme To Lose Weight Naturally

Disclaimer

INDEX

Avoid the Big C – Amazing Programme To Lose
Weight Naturally

Introduction

Avoid the risk of getting the Big C from pills and potions. **In April 2012 the US Food and Drug Administration warned consumers not to take certain Weight Loss Diet Pills" because they contain a suspected cancer-causing agent.** Many such pills are thought to be capable of changing a person's DNA.

It could be argued that many foods also carry health warnings about carcinogenic risk. According to International Science & Technology the following pose the greatest risks of cancer to humans -
Artificial sweeteners
Charred food - burnt popcorn - burnt toast etc.
Excessive alcohol
Farm-raised fish and fish products contain high amounts of PCB's (Polychlorinated Biphenyls)
Fats found in fries and snack chips
(Foods cooked at high temperatures often contain acrylamide)

High salt intake, with spicy foods and smoked food
Meat in general, especially overcooked meat
Sodas
Sugar

The message here is crystal clear. Stay away from Fast Food outlets. So you are down to using natural foods cooked correctly either in the home or in reputable restaurants.

1 Burn Calories and Fats

It's no big secret. It just means changing your lifestyle. If you want to lose weight one of the first things you have to do is burn off the extra calories and fatty deposits. So how to do that is simple. Exercise. The reason you have to exercise is to get the cardiovascular system operating at maximum efficiency.

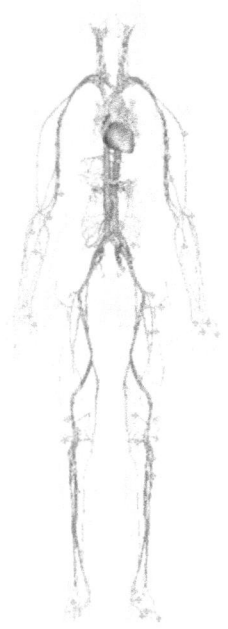

Your lungs, heart and arteries are the most important organs in the cardiovascular system and if they are to remain healthy and operating efficiently they have to be challenged.

You have to exercise. This begs the question – what form of exercise is best? Well of course that depends on you. How much weight do you need to lose? Are you currently mobile? How fit are you? What age are you? You must take all these things into consideration when planning an exercise regime. If you want body beautiful, you're going to have to work hard for it! Some "experts" try to tell us that exercising is counter effective. You burn off fat – you feel hungry – you try a so – called healthy bar (not realising it's full of sugar) and presto all the good work is undone. This is where you will be tested the most. So just drink water and eat fruit after your work out.

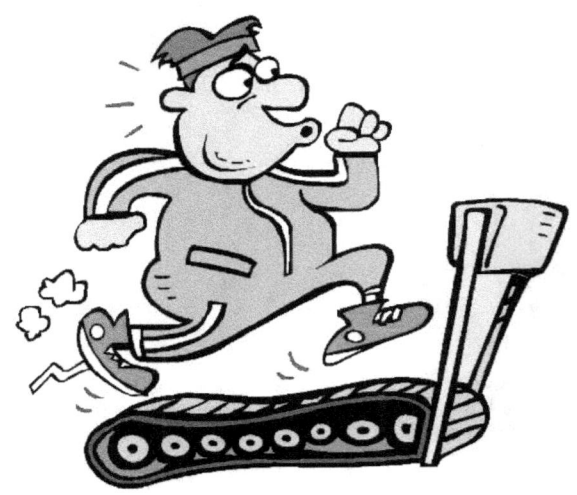

If you are hugely overweight you might be better to join a good gym and have a consultation with a fitness instructor at the outset. He/she will outline a suitable programme for you to follow – such a programme will start with very light exercises that take your physique into account. Remember this is not a quick fix. Bear in mind also that this process can be quite enjoyable. After all you are not alone. You will see many other people with the same problem. After your exercising activity is complete you will be entitled to relax in the Jacuzzi. It's often a great place to start up a conversation! Sharing with other people who have the same problems as you can be helpful in your efforts to combat the fat.

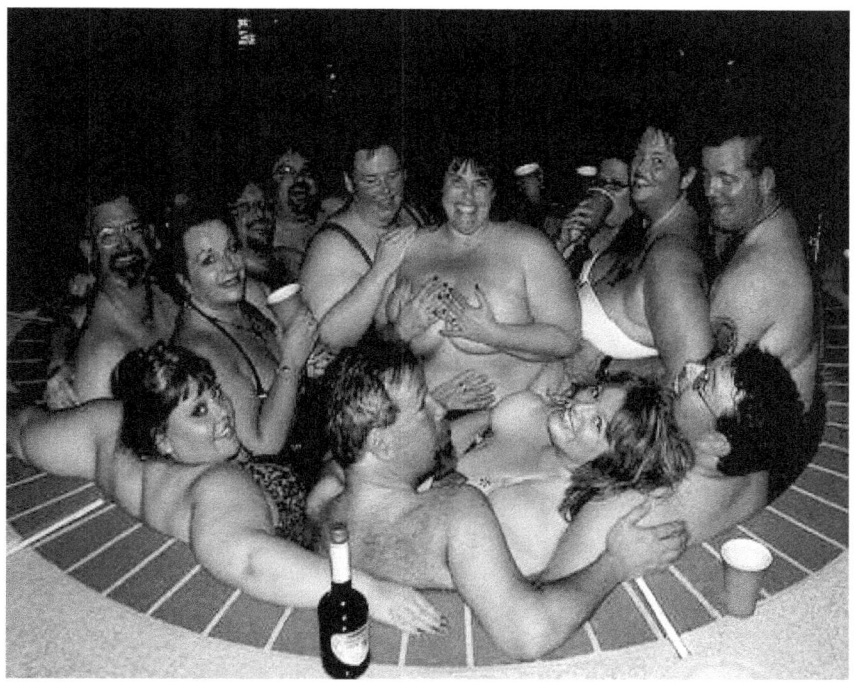

If you are youngish and not grossly overweight then there are many forms of exercise that might appeal to you e.g. walking, running, cycling, swimming, horse riding, yoga, dancing, boxing, skiing, skating, snowboarding, wind surfing, sailing, canoeing, kayaking, climbing, mountaineering, football, basketball, hockey, ice- hockey, athletics, golfing, fishing, backpacking, gardening, fencing, martial arts, handball, badminton, baseball, racquetball, squash, football, soccer, hurling, curling, gymnastics, tennis and volleyball. We included this list so that you might be reminded of all the sports there are out there that might challenge your cardiovascular system!

Of course many of the above mentioned sports/activities are quite suitable for older people too – dancing, walking, swimming, horse riding, sailing, skiing, golfing, fishing, gardening and tennis are the most likely ones.

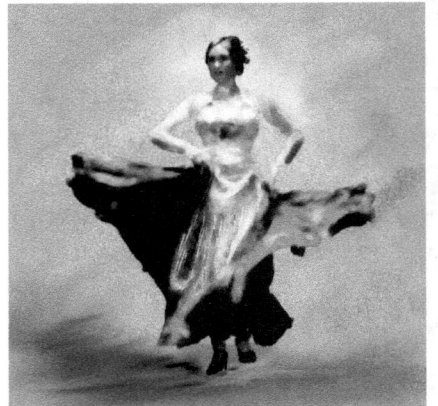

Taking on such sports requires a commitment of your time and sometimes of your money. Take golf for example – if you plan to play golf you should be aware that there are a number of expenses that are unavoidable. You have to buy clubs and golf attire (shoes, wet suit etc.) and you also have to join a club in your locality. Most clubs have a joining fee and an annual subscription which can vary from a few hundred dollars to thousands of dollars. If you plan to play golf you will also have to consider a serious time commitment – generally players allow an entire day for the sport. If you plan to take up any sport be sure to do your research thoroughly.

Walking is perhaps the best option for many people. There is generally a park or promenade within a short distance from most people's homes. Care should be taken to use comfortable walking shoes and suitable clothing that is not too tight fitting. It is also advisable to plan your walking regime. People who are overweight should start with short walks e.g. a mile and build up your distances gradually. After a month it should be possible for the average person to walk about 4 miles without any discomfort.

Of course the walking regime is at the very core of this particular exercise choice (as indeed it is for any exercise you choose). It is very important that you exercise on a regular basis and preferably at the same time every day you do it. Ideally you should exercise every single day. In no time at all you will feel fitter and more energetic.

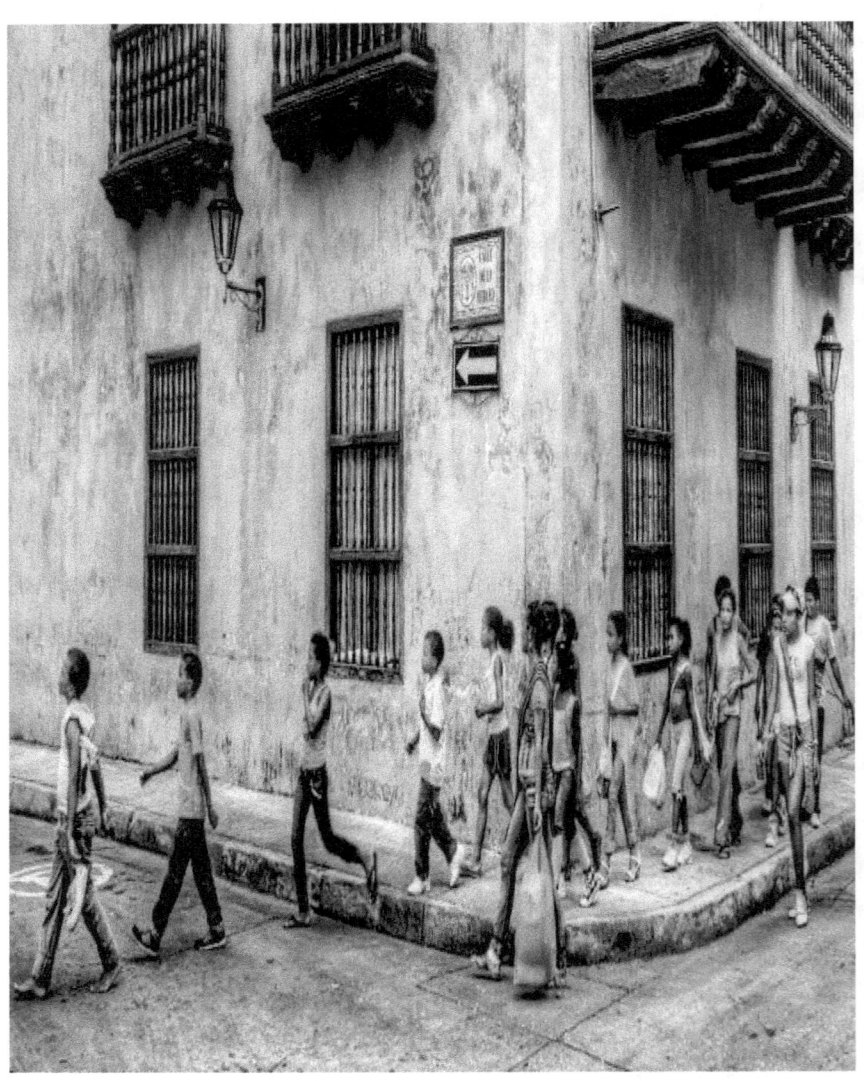

8

2 Design and follow a healthy diet to reduce fat fast.

You are the best person to design your own healthy diet. After all you know best what foods you enjoy and what foods you dislike. Perhaps the best approach might be to write down all the foods you like – those you perceive are good for you and those you think are bad. It would be impossible for us to attempt to list all the foods here that would include all different ethnic dishes. The list would run into many thousands of dishes. So you are the best person to do this particular exercise. The best place to start would be with all the foods you have eaten over the last couple of months.

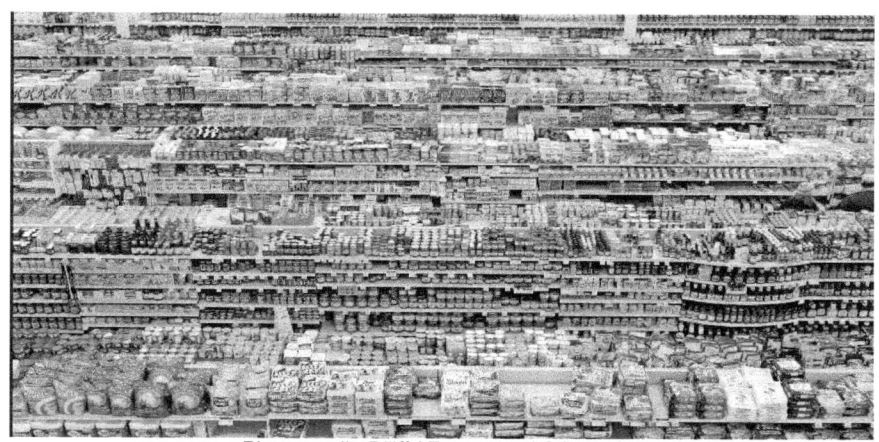

Photo credit: Diliff / Foter.com / CC BY-SA

So how do you know which foods are 'bad' for you? Regardless of the ethnicity of the dishes it is possible to get a good idea.

- **High Sugar Content** - If the food has a high sugar content then it is most likely very bad for anyone trying to lose weight.

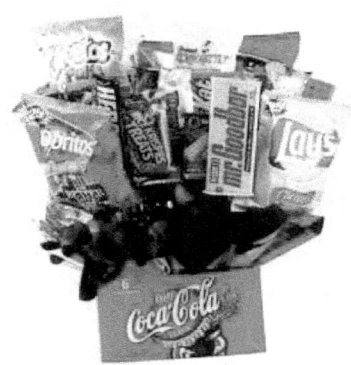

- **High Fat Content** - Likewise a high fat content in the food would indicate that it is not good for you.

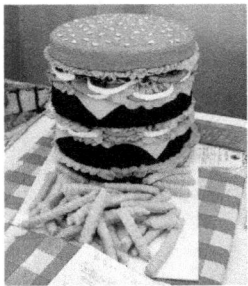

Photo credit: bunchofpants / Foter.com / CC BY-NC-SA

- **High Sodium Content** - Any food with a high sodium content should go on your 'bad' list too.
- **Red meat** - Some studies purport to show that constantly eating red meat can lead to diabetes, heart disease and cancer, all of which can be fatal. Scientists aren't sure exactly what makes red meat so dangerous, but the suspects include the iron and saturated fat in beef, pork and lamb, the nitrates used to preserve them, and the chemicals created by high-temperature cooking.

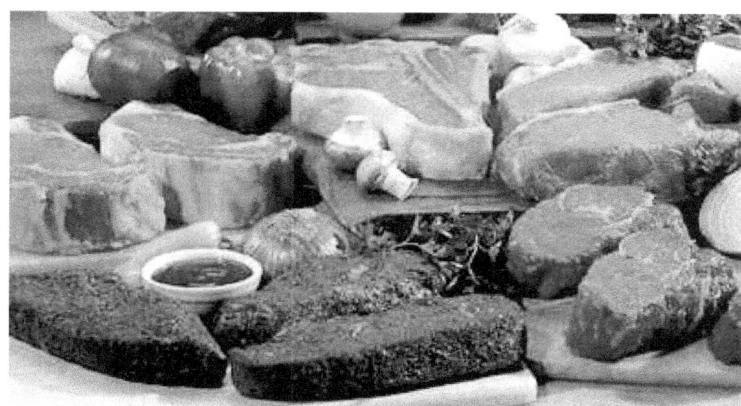

- **Pork** – Pork is not really classified as a red meat but care should be taken if traceability is an issue. Pork tends to be high in fat content so it would be wise to reduce the intake of pork products.

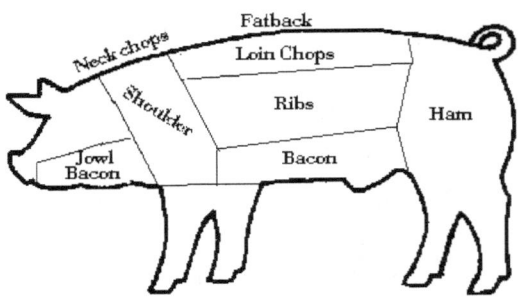

- **Fish** would appear, on the surface at any rate, to be one of the better types of food. Health Guidance for Better Health carried an article recently and this is what they said

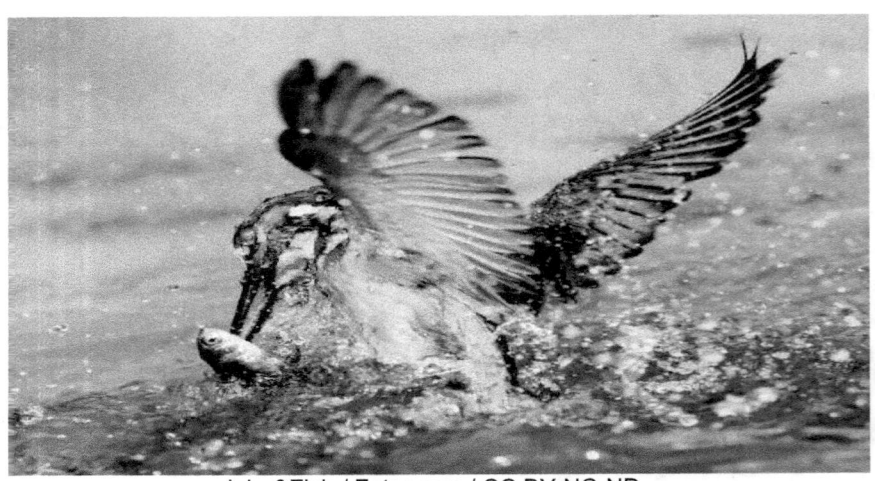

- *Firstly fish oils can be used as an anti inflammatory and can improve your body's inflammatory responses. This means that conditions such as prostatitis, arthritis, cystitis (and pretty much anything ending in 'tis') will be far less painful and uncomfortable. Further to this Omega 3 fatty acids have many cardiovascular benefits and can help lower cholesterol and blood pressure while increasing the 'good' HDL cholesterol. This in turn means less chance of a heart attack, stroke or heart disease. With heart disease being one of the major killers in the Western World this can only be a good thing.*

- **Poultry** is another form of protein that is a bit of a mixed bag. Can anyone be quite sure where the chicken came from? That leads to the question about what it was fed. If you could be reasonably sure that the source of the food is reliable then using poultry would be very beneficial in your diet.

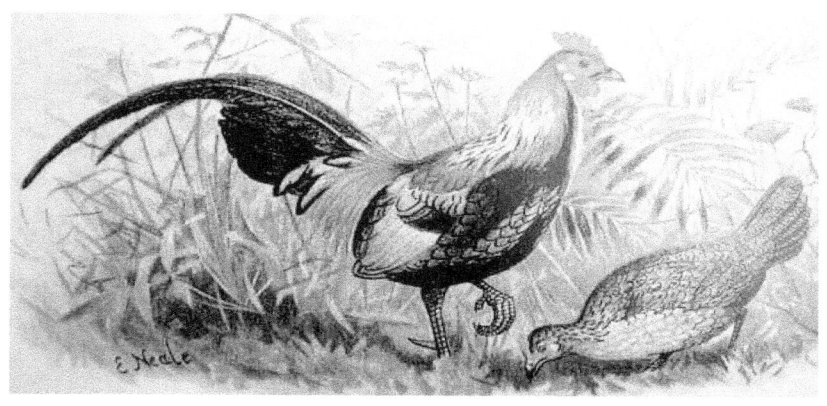

A. O. Hume / Foter.com / Public Domain Mark 1.0

Dairy Products

Milk, Butter, Spreads, Eggs, Yogurts and Drinks Made from Milk are generally all high in fat so eat or drink those products sparingly if you are serious about losing weight.

Nuts

Unfortunately nuts too tend to have a high fat content but the jury is out on whether nuts will actually put on weight. Studies have shown that almond nuts in particular actually contribute to a slight weight loss. Avoid nuts packaged or roasted in oil; instead, eat them raw or dry roasted

3 Lose Weight by eating Vegetables?

Sure you will lose weight if you go on a veggie diet. *Vegan diets tend to be higher in dietary fibre, magnesium, folic acid, vitamin C, vitamin E, iron, and phytochemicals, and lower in calories, saturated fat, cholesterol, long-chain omega-3 fatty acids, vitamin D, calcium, zinc, and vitamin B12. Because uncontaminated plant foods do not provide vitamin B12 (which is produced by microorganisms such as bacteria), researchers agree that vegans should eat foods fortified with B12 or take a daily supplement(Wikipedia)*

The variety and range of vegetables used by humans today is just quite incredible. There are in fact thousands of vegetables that are commonly used in different parts of the world.

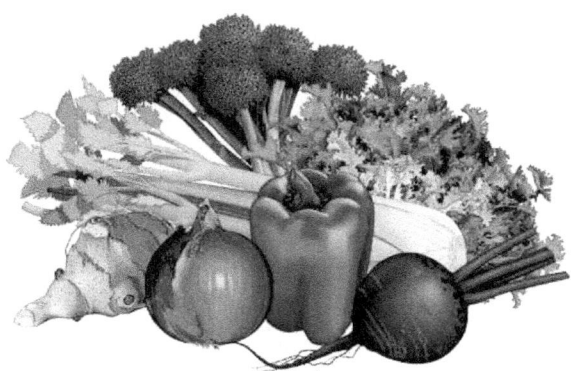

However most of them are derived from some main families of vegetables namely:- Bulb Vegetables, Fruit Vegetables, Inflorescent Vegetables, Leaf Vegetables, Root Vegetables, Stalk Vegetables and Tuber

Vegetables. See the comprehensive list of the main types of vegetables in each category in the table below.

Organic Vegetables are thought by many people to pose less of a risk to people than vegetables grown on farms that use pesticides and sprays but there is no definitive study yet to prove this. The American Cancer Society has said *"whether organic foods carry a lower risk of cancer because they are less likely to be contaminated by compounds that might cause cancer is largely unknown"* but *"vegetables, fruits, and whole grains should form the central part of a person's diet, regardless of whether they are grown conventionally or organically"*

Bulb	Fruit Veg	Inflorescent	Leaf
Chives	Avocados	Artichokes	Arugula
Garlic	Chayote	Broccoli	Brussels sprouts
Leeks	Cucumber	Broccoli rabe	Cabbage
Onions	Eggplant	Cauliflower	Chicory
Scallions	Okra		Chinese cabbage
Shallots	Olives		Collards
Water chestnut	Peppers		Cress
	Squash		Dandelion nettles
	Tomatoes		Endive
	Tomatillos		Lamb's lettuce
			Lettuce
			Nasturtium
			Purslane
			Radicchio
			Savoy
			Sea kale
			Sorrel
			Spinach

Check out these reference tables for ideas

Root	Stalk	Tuber
Beets Burdock Carrots Celeriac Malanga Parsnips Radishes Rutabaga Salsify Turnips	Asparagus Bamboo Cardoon Celery Chard Fiddlehead Fennel Kohlrabi	Cassava Crosne Jerusalem artichoke Jicama Kumara Potato Sweet potato Taro Yam

4 Carbohydrates

Here is a quick lesson about carbohydrates which are essential to maintain life. Carbohydrates are organic compounds that consist only of carbon, hydrogen and oxygen. There are 'good' carbohydrates and 'bad' carbohydrates. We already mentioned one of the 'bad' ones – sugar. Other 'baddies' include white flour, white bread, white rice, white pasta, sweets, candies, processed breakfast cereals, fizzy drinks and refined sugar. The 'good' carbs are vegetables, wholegrain, beans, oats, oatmeal, brown rice, yams, lentils and fruits.

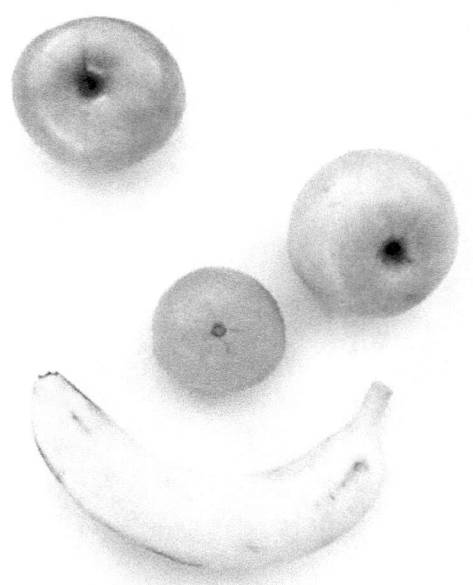

5 Beverages

It might be best to address the question of Alcoholic Drink first. Moderation is the key to all human appetites. Drink in moderation is ok. So what is moderation?

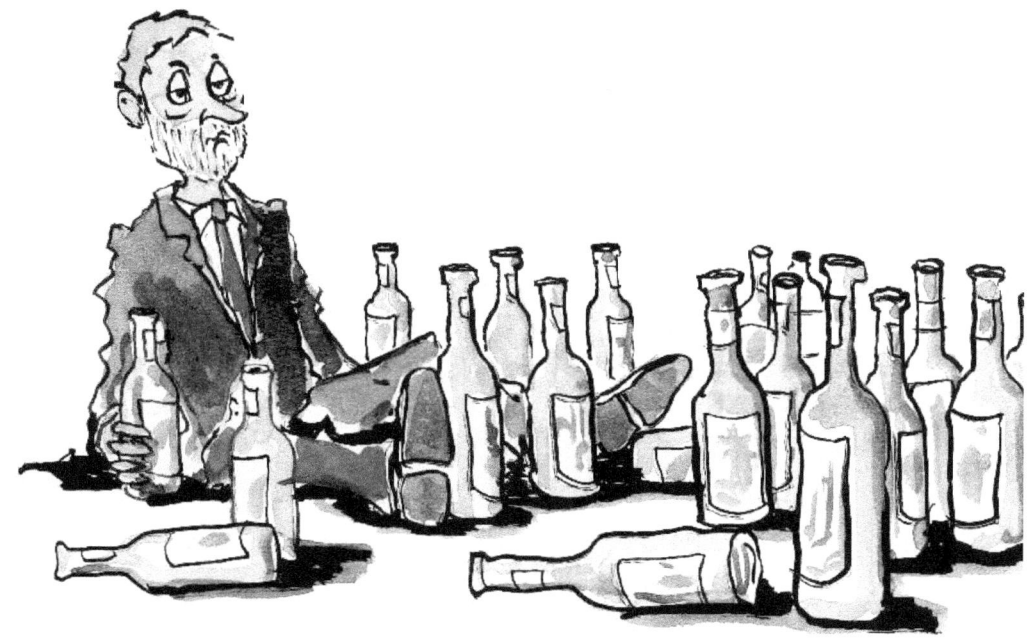

According to the best authorities **Men** should drink no more than 21 units of alcohol per week, four units or less in any one day, and they should have at least two days a week alcohol-free.

Women should drink no more than 14 units of alcohol per week, three units or less in any one day, and have at least two days a week alcohol-free.

Alcoholic Drink	Alcohol Volume	Measure Served	Units of Alcohol
Wine	14%	Small Glass (125 ml.)	1½
Port or Sherry	20%	Standard (50ml.)	1
Spirits	40%	Standard ½Glass(35 ml.)	1½
Beer/Lager	3-4 %	Half Pint (450 ml)	1
Cider	3-4 %	Half Pint (240 ml)	1

Does Alcohol put on weight? Recent studies have found that older people tend to put on abdominal fat if they drink to excess. This is not particularly the case with younger people but if they gorge themselves on all the wrong foods at the same time they will definitely put on belly fat. Many alcoholics are thin and scrawny but that is because they don't eat much – their focus is on getting alcohol into their systems. Alcohol adds calories into a person's diet, can interfere with hormones and can stimulate appetite, leading to even more calories consumed.

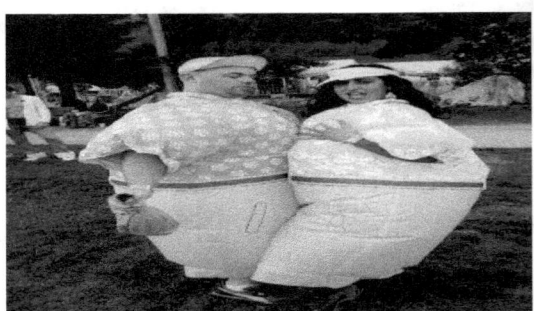

noah.w / Foter.com / CC BY-NC-SA

Coffee: Coffee is an institution in America. It would seem that everyone drinks coffee. Most people drink coffee with sugar added and with milk or cream. A huge proportion of the population appears to drink on average more than 3 cups per day. Of course some people drink a lot more. People who drink a lot of coffee tend to be fatter. It is thought that 2 cups of coffee per day is OK but with no sugar added and very little milk.

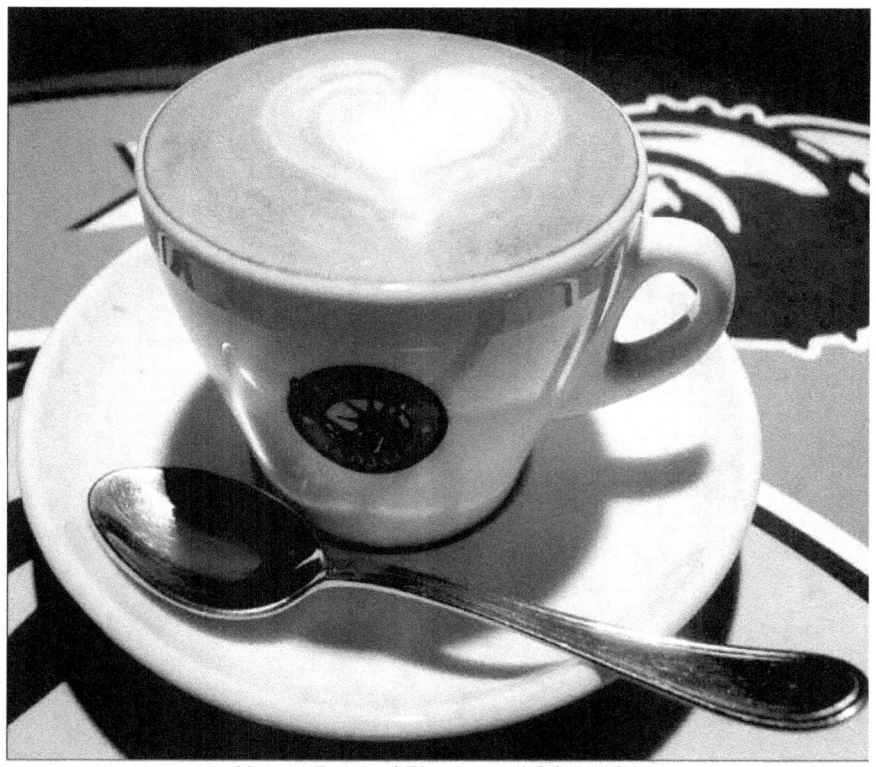

Ahmed Rabea / Foter.com / CC BY-SA

Tea: Tea is not known to be a factor in weight gain, but like coffee tea is often taken with sugar and milk and they will definitely lead to weight gain. A better option might be to take herbal or green tea.

Milk: Milk is fattening. Even skimmed milk still has residues of fat at either 1 or 2 per cent. Buttermilk has very little fat residue. The use of skimmed milk or buttermilk is acceptable in a weight loss programme.

Soft Drinks: If you want to lose weight you would be best advised to avoid soft drinks – many of them have high levels of sugar or sodium or both.

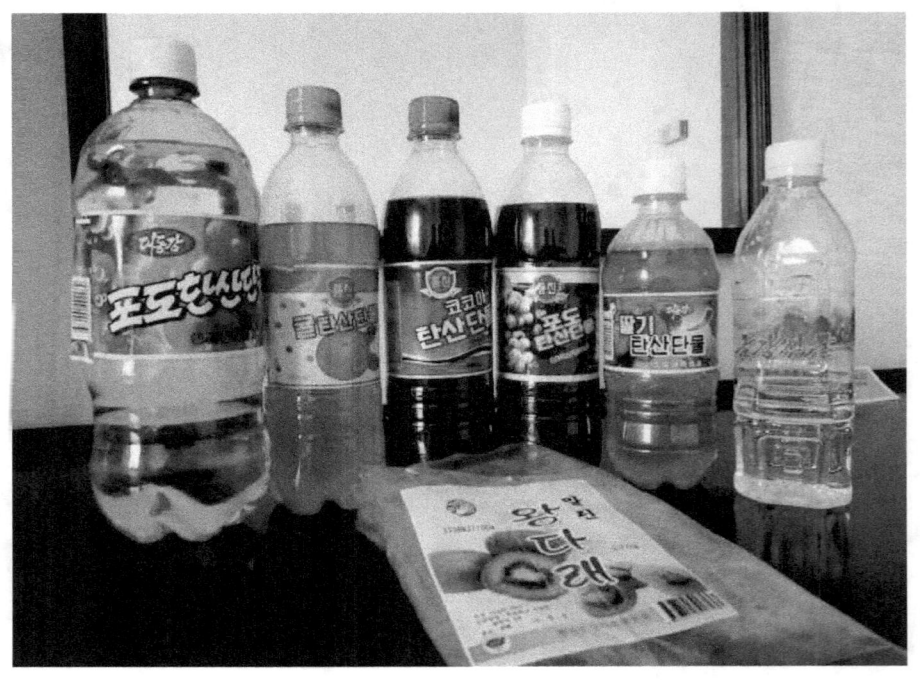

6 Amazing Programme

Here it is – The Amazing Programme that will see you lose weight fast.

FIRST: Set up an exercise regime that will challenge your cardiovascular system. There is no use walking 4 miles at a snail's pace. Your lungs must be expanded and your pulse rate increased. Depending on yourself you must decide what form of exercise to do. But if you want to lose weight naturally and become a healthy human being you have to exercise. Sorry folks, there is no other way! And do remember that your exercise regime must be carried on a daily basis or at worst every second day but we highly recommend exercising daily. You could combine different exercise regimes. For example you might decide to swim on one day and walk or jog on another and you might play golf on Sundays.

SECOND: You must decide on a diet. Here is a diet that works.

Breakfast: Portion of Fresh Fruit e.g. ¼Pineapple
Porridge with Skim Milk
1 Slice of Brown Bread with Honey
1 Cup of Coffee, Weak Tea or Herbal Tea

Lunch:	Portion of Fresh Fruit
	Salad (light dressing) with Rye Crisbread
	Tuna/Sardines/Chicken with Rye Crisbread
	1 Slice of Brown Bread with Honey
	1 Cup of Coffee, Weak Tea or Herbal Tea

Dinner:	Fresh Fish/Chicken with Veg & Potato
	Glass of Wine
	Glass of Water
	1 Slice Homemade Tea Brack

It is permissible to put a very small amount of low fat spread on your Brown Bread, Crispbread and Tea Brack. Occasionally you might try Beef or Lamb for your Dinner but be sure it is lean meat.

And absolutely no desserts – other than the Tea Brack.

THIRD: Drink in moderation as per the suggestions above

That's it folks. It's really simple. Keep it simple and it will work.

Stick to simple plain foods and simple drinks. Do not snack, but if you must, take something very simple e.g. fresh fruit, nuts or a slice of brown bread with honey and a cup of herbal tea. Exercise every day preferably at the same times. Eat at the same times. Drink plenty of water.

And stay away from pills that promise weight loss.

Thank you for buying this ebook and I know that if you follow the suggestions to the letter you will have success-naturally.

Good luck with your weight loss programme.

Jim Finnegan